My Kefir Log

AF808786

Right Track Publishing

Olathe, KS

My Kefir Log
The Fervent Fermenter Series

Published by Right Track Publishing in 2017

righttrackpublishing.com

The information provided in this publication is for educational and record-keeping purposes only, and is not intended to replace professional medical or nutritional advice.

ISBN: 978-0-9913371-3-2

Kefir Basics

Kefir is a healthy fermented drink traditionally made from milk. It has similar characteristics to yogurt and is vitamin rich, along with minerals, enzymes, and probiotics.

Kefir originated in the area of the Caucasus Mountains many centuries ago. We might never know how exactly it began, but we do know that the ancients often used fermentation as a method of preserving foods.

Buying pre-bottled kefir can be expensive if you plan on drinking the beverage regularly. Making your own is a fun, simple, and cost-effective alternative.

You will need:

- ✔ Pint or quart-size glass container
- ✔ Milk (cow, goat, sheep) (whole or 2%)
- ✔ Kefir grains
- ✔ Cloth or coffee filters for cover
- ✔ Spoon
- ✔ Strainer

For best results, it's recommended you follow the detailed directions from your favorite kefir book or website. Always take proper precautions for sanitary food preparation before starting your kefir.

Ingredients:

1 quart of milk

1 tablespoon of active kefir grains

Kefir grains can be purchased online from reputable suppliers (look for good ratings and reviews).

Put the kefir grains into a quart glass jar, fill with milk, leaving 1/2 to 1-inch space at top. Cover with coffee filter or clean cloth and secure with a rubber band. Place jar on counter out of direct sunlight. Ideal room temperature should be between 72 and 80-degrees.

Kefir takes 24 to 48 hours to ferment, but most people like to keep it on the shorter end. The longer it ferments, the more tart it will be. When the kefir is ready, strain out the kefir grains to use for the next batch. The kefir is then ready for drinking or chilling in the refrigerator.

At this point the kefir is ready for a second ferment if you want to add flavoring, such as: cinnamon, vanilla, pumpkin pie spice, cocoa, or fruit. Let the kefir sit with the flavoring for up to six hours. Remove pieces of fruit to prevent the kefir from separating or carbonating (it isn't bad if it does). Chill the kefir to enjoy it cold. Many home-fermenters like the second fermentation because the amount of probiotics and vitamins increase, and it taste smoother as well.

The process is slightly different for non-dairy. For further information on kefir, or instructions on how to make **non-dairy kefir**, please check out the following resources!

The resources below are great go-to's for beginners:

Websites

thekitchn.com/how-to-make-milk-kefir-cooking-lessons-from-the-kitchn-202022

kombuchakamp.com/milk-kefir-recipes-and-tips

culturesforhealth.com/learn/recipe/milk-kefir/coconut-milk-kefir-recipe/

Books

Delicious Probiotic Drinks: 75 Recipes for Kombucha, Kefir, Ginger Beer, and Other Naturally Fermented Drinks
by Julia Mueller

Water Kefir Mastery: Complete Guidebook to Brewing and Mastering Water Kefir (Health and Wellness Mastery Series)
by Dylan Barnes

Details

Type: ☐ Dairy ☐ Non-Dairy

Vessel Size ________ Room Temp ______

Start Date / Time ________________________

Milk Type ________________________

Other liquid ________________________

☐ 24-hours / Flavor ______________________

☐ Total hours ____ Flavor _______________

Harvest Date / Time ______________________

Flavorings Added ________________________

____

Hours for Second Ferment:

1 2 3 4 5 6 Other ____

Notes:

Details

Type: ☐ Dairy ☐ Non-Dairy

Vessel Size ________ Room Temp ______

Start Date / Time ________________________

Milk Type ________________________

Other liquid ________________________

☐ 24-hours / Flavor ______________________

☐ Total hours _____ Flavor _______________

Harvest Date / Time ________________________

Flavorings Added _________________________

____

Hours for Second Ferment:

1 2 3 4 5 6 Other _____

Notes:

Details

Type: ☐ Dairy ☐ Non-Dairy

Vessel Size ________ Room Temp ______

Start Date / Time ________________________

Milk Type ________________________

Other liquid ________________________

☐ 24-hours / Flavor ______________________

☐ Total hours _____ Flavor _______________

Harvest Date / Time ________________________

Flavorings Added __________________________

____

Hours for Second Ferment:

1 2 3 4 5 6 Other _____

Notes:

Details

Type: ☐ Dairy ☐ Non-Dairy

Vessel Size ________ Room Temp ______

Start Date / Time ________________________

Milk Type ________________________

Other liquid ________________________

☐ 24-hours / Flavor ______________________

☐ Total hours _____ Flavor _______________

Harvest Date / Time ________________________

Flavorings Added __________________________

____

Hours for Second Ferment:

1 2 3 4 5 6 Other _____

Notes:

Details

Type: ☐ Dairy ☐ Non-Dairy

Vessel Size ________ Room Temp ______

Start Date / Time ________________________

Milk Type ________________________

Other liquid ________________________

☐ 24-hours / Flavor ______________________

☐ Total hours _____ Flavor _______________

Harvest Date / Time ________________________

Flavorings Added __________________________

____

Hours for Second Ferment:

1 2 3 4 5 6 Other _____

Notes:

Details

Type: ☐ Dairy ☐ Non-Dairy

Vessel Size ________ Room Temp ______

Start Date / Time ________________________

Milk Type ________________________

Other liquid ________________________

☐ 24-hours / Flavor ______________________

☐ Total hours _____ Flavor _______________

Harvest Date / Time ________________________

Flavorings Added __________________________

____

Hours for Second Ferment:

1 2 3 4 5 6 Other _____

Notes:

Details

Type: ☐ Dairy ☐ Non-Dairy

Vessel Size ________ Room Temp _____

Start Date / Time ________________________

Milk Type ________________________

Other liquid ________________________

☐ 24-hours / Flavor ______________________

☐ Total hours ____ Flavor _______________

Harvest Date / Time ______________________

Flavorings Added _________________________

____

Hours for Second Ferment:

1 2 3 4 5 6 Other ____

Notes:

Details

Type: ☐ Dairy ☐ Non-Dairy

Vessel Size ________ Room Temp ______

Start Date / Time

Milk Type

Other liquid

☐ 24-hours / Flavor ______________________

☐ Total hours _____ Flavor _______________

Harvest Date / Time

Flavorings Added _________________________

____

Hours for Second Ferment:

1 2 3 4 5 6 Other _____

Notes:

Details

Type: ☐ Dairy ☐ Non-Dairy

Vessel Size ________ Room Temp ______

Start Date / Time ________________________

Milk Type ________________________

Other liquid ________________________

☐ 24-hours / Flavor ______________________

☐ Total hours ____ Flavor _______________

Harvest Date / Time ________________________

Flavorings Added __________________________

____

Hours for Second Ferment:

1 2 3 4 5 6 Other ____

Notes:

Details

Type: ☐ Dairy ☐ Non-Dairy

Vessel Size ________ Room Temp ______

Start Date / Time ________________________

Milk Type ________________________

Other liquid ________________________

☐ 24-hours / Flavor ______________________

☐ Total hours _____ Flavor ________________

Harvest Date / Time ________________________

Flavorings Added __________________________

____

Hours for Second Ferment:

1 2 3 4 5 6 Other _____

Notes:

Details

Type: ☐ Dairy ☐ Non-Dairy

Vessel Size ________ Room Temp ______

Start Date / Time ________________________

Milk Type ________________________

Other liquid ________________________

☐ 24-hours / Flavor ______________________

☐ Total hours _____ Flavor _______________

Harvest Date / Time ________________________

Flavorings Added __________________________

____

Hours for Second Ferment:

1 2 3 4 5 6 Other _____

Notes:

Details

Type: ☐ Dairy ☐ Non-Dairy

Vessel Size ________ Room Temp ______

Start Date / Time ________________________

Milk Type ________________________

Other liquid ________________________

☐ 24-hours / Flavor ______________________

☐ Total hours _____ Flavor _______________

Harvest Date / Time ________________________

Flavorings Added __________________________

____

Hours for Second Ferment:

1 2 3 4 5 6 Other _____

Notes:

Details

Type: ☐ Dairy ☐ Non-Dairy

Vessel Size ________ Room Temp ______

Start Date / Time ________________________

Milk Type ________________________

Other liquid ________________________

☐ 24-hours / Flavor ______________________

☐ Total hours _____ Flavor _______________

Harvest Date / Time ______________________

Flavorings Added __________________________

____

Hours for Second Ferment:

1 2 3 4 5 6 Other _____

Notes:

Details

Type: ☐ Dairy ☐ Non-Dairy

Vessel Size ________ Room Temp ______

Start Date / Time ________________________

Milk Type ________________________

Other liquid ________________________

☐ 24-hours / Flavor ______________________

☐ Total hours ____ Flavor _______________

Harvest Date / Time ________________________

Flavorings Added __________________________

____

Hours for Second Ferment:

1 2 3 4 5 6 Other ____

Notes:

Details

Type: ☐ Dairy ☐ Non-Dairy

Vessel Size ________ Room Temp ______

Start Date / Time ______________________

Milk Type ______________________

Other liquid ______________________

☐ 24-hours / Flavor ______________________

☐ Total hours _____ Flavor ________________

Harvest Date / Time ______________________

Flavorings Added ___________________________

____

Hours for Second Ferment:

1 2 3 4 5 6 Other _____

Notes:

Details

Type: ☐ Dairy ☐ Non-Dairy

Vessel Size ________ Room Temp ______

Start Date / Time

Milk Type

Other liquid

☐ 24-hours / Flavor ______________________

☐ Total hours _____ Flavor _______________

Harvest Date / Time

Flavorings Added __________________________

____

Hours for Second Ferment:

1 2 3 4 5 6 Other _____

Notes:

Details

Type: ☐ Dairy ☐ Non-Dairy

Vessel Size ________ Room Temp ______

Start Date / Time ________________________

Milk Type ________________________

Other liquid ________________________

☐ 24-hours / Flavor ______________________

☐ Total hours _____ Flavor _______________

Harvest Date / Time ______________________

Flavorings Added _________________________

____

Hours for Second Ferment:

1 2 3 4 5 6 Other _____

Notes:

Details

Type: ☐ Dairy ☐ Non-Dairy

Vessel Size ________ Room Temp ______

Start Date / Time ________________________

Milk Type ________________________

Other liquid ________________________

☐ 24-hours / Flavor ______________________

☐ Total hours _____ Flavor _______________

Harvest Date / Time ________________________

Flavorings Added __________________________

____

Hours for Second Ferment:

1 2 3 4 5 6 Other _____

Notes:

Details

Type: ☐ Dairy ☐ Non-Dairy

Vessel Size ________ Room Temp ______

Start Date / Time ________________________

Milk Type ________________________

Other liquid ________________________

☐ 24-hours / Flavor ______________________

☐ Total hours _____ Flavor _______________

Harvest Date / Time ________________________

Flavorings Added __________________________

____

Hours for Second Ferment:

1 2 3 4 5 6 Other _____

Notes:

Details

Type: ☐ Dairy ☐ Non-Dairy

Vessel Size ________ Room Temp ______

Start Date / Time

Milk Type

Other liquid

☐ 24-hours / Flavor ______________________

☐ Total hours _____ Flavor _______________

Harvest Date / Time

Flavorings Added _________________________

____

Hours for Second Ferment:

1 2 3 4 5 6 Other _____

Notes:

Details

Type: ☐ Dairy ☐ Non-Dairy

Vessel Size ________ Room Temp ______

Start Date / Time

Milk Type

Other liquid

☐ 24-hours / Flavor ______________________

☐ Total hours ____ Flavor _______________

Harvest Date / Time

Flavorings Added __________________________

____

Hours for Second Ferment:

1 2 3 4 5 6 Other ____

Notes:

Details

Type: ☐ Dairy ☐ Non-Dairy

Vessel Size ________ Room Temp _____

Start Date / Time ________________________

Milk Type ________________________

Other liquid ________________________

☐ 24-hours / Flavor ______________________

☐ Total hours ____ Flavor ______________

Harvest Date / Time ______________________

Flavorings Added _________________________

____

Hours for Second Ferment:

1 2 3 4 5 6 Other ____

Notes:

Details

Type: ☐ Dairy ☐ Non-Dairy

Vessel Size ________ Room Temp ______

Start Date / Time ________________________

Milk Type ________________________

Other liquid ________________________

☐ 24-hours / Flavor ______________________

☐ Total hours ____ Flavor _______________

Harvest Date / Time ________________________

Flavorings Added ___________________________

____

Hours for Second Ferment:

1 2 3 4 5 6 Other ____

Notes:

Details

Type: ☐ Dairy ☐ Non-Dairy

Vessel Size ________ Room Temp ______

Start Date / Time ________________________

Milk Type ________________________

Other liquid ________________________

☐ 24-hours / Flavor ______________________

☐ Total hours _____ Flavor _______________

Harvest Date / Time ________________________

Flavorings Added __________________________

____

Hours for Second Ferment:

1 2 3 4 5 6 Other _____

Notes:

Details

Type: ☐ Dairy ☐ Non-Dairy

Vessel Size ________ Room Temp ______

Start Date / Time

Milk Type

Other liquid

☐ 24-hours / Flavor ______________________

☐ Total hours ____ Flavor _______________

Harvest Date / Time

Flavorings Added _________________________

____

Hours for Second Ferment:

1 2 3 4 5 6 Other ____

Notes:

Details

Type: ☐ Dairy ☐ Non-Dairy

Vessel Size _______ Room Temp _____

Start Date / Time

Milk Type

Other liquid

☐ 24-hours / Flavor ___________________

☐ Total hours ____ Flavor _____________

Harvest Date / Time

Flavorings Added ______________________

____

Hours for Second Ferment:

1 2 3 4 5 6 Other ____

Notes:

Details

Type: ☐ Dairy ☐ Non-Dairy

Vessel Size _______ Room Temp _____

Start Date / Time ____________________

Milk Type ____________________

Other liquid ____________________

☐ 24-hours / Flavor ____________________

☐ Total hours ____ Flavor ______________

Harvest Date / Time ____________________

Flavorings Added ______________________

____

Hours for Second Ferment:

1 2 3 4 5 6 Other ____

Notes:

Details

Type: ☐ Dairy ☐ Non-Dairy

Vessel Size ________ Room Temp ______

Start Date / Time ________________________

Milk Type ________________________

Other liquid ________________________

☐ 24-hours / Flavor ______________________

☐ Total hours _____ Flavor _______________

Harvest Date / Time ________________________

Flavorings Added _________________________

____

Hours for Second Ferment:

1 2 3 4 5 6 Other _____

Notes:

Details

Type: ☐ Dairy ☐ Non-Dairy

Vessel Size _______ Room Temp _____

Start Date / Time ____________________

Milk Type ____________________

Other liquid ____________________

☐ 24-hours / Flavor ____________________

☐ Total hours ____ Flavor _____________

Harvest Date / Time ____________________

Flavorings Added ______________________

____

Hours for Second Ferment:

1 2 3 4 5 6 Other ____

Notes:

Details

Type: ☐ Dairy ☐ Non-Dairy

Vessel Size ________ Room Temp ______

Start Date / Time ________________________

Milk Type ________________________

Other liquid ________________________

☐ 24-hours / Flavor ______________________

☐ Total hours _____ Flavor _______________

Harvest Date / Time ________________________

Flavorings Added __________________________

____

Hours for Second Ferment:

1 2 3 4 5 6 Other _____

Notes:

Details

Type: ☐ Dairy ☐ Non-Dairy

Vessel Size ________ Room Temp ______

Start Date / Time ________________________

Milk Type ________________________

Other liquid ________________________

☐ 24-hours / Flavor ______________________

☐ Total hours _____ Flavor _______________

Harvest Date / Time ______________________

Flavorings Added __________________________

____

Hours for Second Ferment:

1 2 3 4 5 6 Other _____

Notes:

Details

Type: ☐ Dairy ☐ Non-Dairy

Vessel Size _______ Room Temp _____

Start Date / Time ____________________

Milk Type ____________________

Other liquid ____________________

☐ 24-hours / Flavor ____________________

☐ Total hours ____ Flavor _____________

Harvest Date / Time ____________________

Flavorings Added ______________________

____

Hours for Second Ferment:

1 2 3 4 5 6 Other ____

Notes:

Details

Type: ☐ Dairy ☐ Non-Dairy

Vessel Size _______ Room Temp _____

Start Date / Time

Milk Type

Other liquid

☐ 24-hours / Flavor ___________________

☐ Total hours ____ Flavor _____________

Harvest Date / Time

Flavorings Added ______________________

____

Hours for Second Ferment:

1 2 3 4 5 6 Other ____

Notes:

Details

Type: ☐ Dairy ☐ Non-Dairy

Vessel Size ________ Room Temp ______

Start Date / Time ________________________

Milk Type ________________________

Other liquid ________________________

☐ 24-hours / Flavor ______________________

☐ Total hours _____ Flavor _______________

Harvest Date / Time ________________________

Flavorings Added __________________________

____

Hours for Second Ferment:

1 2 3 4 5 6 Other _____

Notes:

Details

Type: ☐ Dairy ☐ Non-Dairy

Vessel Size _______ Room Temp _____

Start Date / Time

Milk Type

Other liquid

☐ 24-hours / Flavor ___________________

☐ Total hours ____ Flavor _____________

Harvest Date / Time

Flavorings Added ______________________

____

Hours for Second Ferment:

1 2 3 4 5 6 Other ____

Notes:

Details

Type: ☐ Dairy ☐ Non-Dairy

Vessel Size ________ Room Temp ______

Start Date / Time ________________________

Milk Type ________________________

Other liquid ________________________

☐ 24-hours / Flavor ______________________

☐ Total hours _____ Flavor _______________

Harvest Date / Time ________________________

Flavorings Added __________________________

____

Hours for Second Ferment:

1 2 3 4 5 6 Other _____

Notes:

Details

Type: ☐ Dairy ☐ Non-Dairy

Vessel Size ________ Room Temp ______

Start Date / Time ________________________

Milk Type ________________________

Other liquid ________________________

☐ 24-hours / Flavor ______________________

☐ Total hours _____ Flavor _______________

Harvest Date / Time ________________________

Flavorings Added _________________________

____

Hours for Second Ferment:

1 2 3 4 5 6 Other _____

Notes:

Details

Type: ☐ Dairy ☐ Non-Dairy

Vessel Size _______ Room Temp _____

Start Date / Time

Milk Type

Other liquid

☐ 24-hours / Flavor ___________________

☐ Total hours ____ Flavor _____________

Harvest Date / Time

Flavorings Added ______________________

____

Hours for Second Ferment:

1 2 3 4 5 6 Other ____

Notes:

Details

Type: ☐ Dairy ☐ Non-Dairy

Vessel Size ________ Room Temp ______

Start Date / Time ________________________

Milk Type ________________________

Other liquid ________________________

☐ 24-hours / Flavor ______________________

☐ Total hours _____ Flavor _______________

Harvest Date / Time ________________________

Flavorings Added __________________________

____

Hours for Second Ferment:

1 2 3 4 5 6 Other _____

Notes:

Details

Type: ☐ Dairy ☐ Non-Dairy

Vessel Size ________ Room Temp ______

Start Date / Time ________________________

Milk Type ________________________

Other liquid ________________________

☐ 24-hours / Flavor ______________________

☐ Total hours _____ Flavor _______________

Harvest Date / Time ______________________

Flavorings Added __________________________

____

Hours for Second Ferment:

1 2 3 4 5 6 Other _____

Notes:

Details

Type: ☐ Dairy ☐ Non-Dairy

Vessel Size _______ Room Temp _____

Start Date / Time ____________________

Milk Type ____________________

Other liquid ____________________

☐ 24-hours / Flavor ____________________

☐ Total hours ____ Flavor _____________

Harvest Date / Time ____________________

Flavorings Added ______________________

____

Hours for Second Ferment:

1 2 3 4 5 6 Other ____

Notes:

Details

Type: ☐ Dairy ☐ Non-Dairy

Vessel Size ________ Room Temp ______

Start Date / Time ________________________

Milk Type ________________________

Other liquid ________________________

☐ 24-hours / Flavor ______________________

☐ Total hours ____ Flavor _______________

Harvest Date / Time ________________________

Flavorings Added __________________________

____

Hours for Second Ferment:

1 2 3 4 5 6 Other ____

Notes:

Details

Type: ☐ Dairy ☐ Non-Dairy

Vessel Size ________ Room Temp ______

Start Date / Time ________________________

Milk Type ________________________

Other liquid ________________________

☐ 24-hours / Flavor ______________________

☐ Total hours _____ Flavor _______________

Harvest Date / Time ________________________

Flavorings Added __________________________

____

Hours for Second Ferment:

1 2 3 4 5 6 Other _____

Notes:

Details

Type: ☐ Dairy ☐ Non-Dairy

Vessel Size ________ Room Temp ______

Start Date / Time ________________________

Milk Type ________________________

Other liquid ________________________

☐ 24-hours / Flavor ______________________

☐ Total hours _____ Flavor _______________

Harvest Date / Time ______________________

Flavorings Added _________________________

____

Hours for Second Ferment:

1 2 3 4 5 6 Other _____

Notes:

Details

Type: ☐ Dairy ☐ Non-Dairy

Vessel Size ________ Room Temp ______

Start Date / Time ______________________

Milk Type ______________________

Other liquid ______________________

☐ 24-hours / Flavor ______________________

☐ Total hours _____ Flavor _______________

Harvest Date / Time ______________________

Flavorings Added _________________________

____

Hours for Second Ferment:

1 2 3 4 5 6 Other _____

Notes:

Details

Type: ☐ Dairy ☐ Non-Dairy

Vessel Size ________ Room Temp _____

Start Date / Time

Milk Type

Other liquid

☐ 24-hours / Flavor ______________________

☐ Total hours ____ Flavor _______________

Harvest Date / Time

Flavorings Added _________________________

____

Hours for Second Ferment:

1 2 3 4 5 6 Other ____

Notes:

Details

Type: ☐ Dairy ☐ Non-Dairy

Vessel Size _______ Room Temp _____

Start Date / Time ____________________

Milk Type ____________________

Other liquid ____________________

☐ 24-hours / Flavor ____________________

☐ Total hours ____ Flavor _____________

Harvest Date / Time ____________________

Flavorings Added ______________________

____

Hours for Second Ferment:

1 2 3 4 5 6 Other ____

Notes:

Details

Type: ☐ Dairy ☐ Non-Dairy

Vessel Size ________ Room Temp ______

Start Date / Time ________________________

Milk Type ________________________

Other liquid ________________________

☐ 24-hours / Flavor ______________________

☐ Total hours _____ Flavor _______________

Harvest Date / Time ________________________

Flavorings Added __________________________

____

Hours for Second Ferment:

1 2 3 4 5 6 Other _____

Notes:

Details

Type: ☐ Dairy ☐ Non-Dairy

Vessel Size ________ Room Temp ______

Start Date / Time ________________________

Milk Type ________________________

Other liquid ________________________

☐ 24-hours / Flavor ______________________

☐ Total hours _____ Flavor _______________

Harvest Date / Time ______________________

Flavorings Added _________________________

____

Hours for Second Ferment:

1 2 3 4 5 6 Other _____

Notes:

Details

Type: ☐ Dairy ☐ Non-Dairy

Vessel Size ________ Room Temp ______

Start Date / Time ________________________

Milk Type ________________________

Other liquid ________________________

☐ 24-hours / Flavor ______________________

☐ Total hours _____ Flavor _______________

Harvest Date / Time ______________________

Flavorings Added __________________________

____

Hours for Second Ferment:

1 2 3 4 5 6 Other _____

Notes: